AIR FRYER MASTERY

An Easy and Understandable Cookbook Guide to Air Fryer for Beginners

Hollie McCarthy RDN

Introduction

Welcome to the air fryer guide!

The air fryer is one of the most impressive and useful inventions of the decade. With this machine, you can reduce the amount of grease you consume from traditional dishes and snacks such as chicken nuggets and French fries. Goes without saying that cooking time is considerably reduced!

It is a multi-cooker that performs more than functions. The air fryer enables you to cook a wide variety of dishes including meat, fish, eggs, grain, poultry, beans, cakes, yogurt and vegetables etc. What Serves: it exceptional is because you can use different cooking programs such as a steamer, rice cooker, sauté pan, and even a warming pot, thus saving more time, money, and space than buying any other kitchen appliances.

The Air fryer Serves: as a multi-use programmable appliance can help create easy, fast and flavorful recipes with the ability to apply different cooking settings all in one pot. It was developed by Canadian technology experts seeking to be the ultimate kitchen mate, from stir-frying, pressure cooking, slow cooking and yogurt and cake making. It was created to serve as a one-stop shop to allow home cooks prepare a tasty meal with the press of a button. You can cook almost everything in this fryer.

The air fryer uses an ingenious combination of both Directions, differing from the convection oven because heat circulates everywhere (vice rising to the top) through the fan, and not through the turbo because there is typically no heating element in the top of a fryer from where the heat comes out. They use electrical energy to create their heat; a lot of power!

Many people still have their doubts regarding the importance of this machine, and what a healthy alternative it can be. Despite its popularity, in some regions it has not yet reached the peak of its use. It is very likely that in a short time new brands will emerge in other regions and the air fryer will grow in popularity across the nation.

The use of this tool consists of cooking something without boiling the product in oil or fat. At most, the maximum oil needed by the air fryer is a tablespoon, which is used to prevent the food from sticking and forming an overdone crust.

What is an air fryer?

An air fryer works with "fast air technology." This means that there is a highspeed circulation of hot air that cocoons the food you cook.

During this process, the air fryer prepares the food evenly, all the while giving it a "fried" taste and texture without ever actually having to fry anything in grease.

While many people and regions near and far are familiar with this tool, the electric fryer is even crossing the waters. They are even found commonly in Europe and Australia!

The air fryer is similar in concept to a convection oven or a turbo grill, although the fryer still differs slightly from both appliances. Convection ovens and turbo broilers depend on different heating Directions and are often larger and bulkier appliances to use when cooking your food.

In this book, we will explore the variety of easy delicious dishes you can cook with your air fryer. We will explore a wide variety of dishes, from breakfast to dinner, soups to stews, desserts to appetizers, meat to beef, side dishes to vegetables and use a healthy ingredient in the process. The vast majority of the recipes can be prepared and served in less than 45 minutes. Each recipe is written with the exact cooking Directions and ingredients required to prepare dishes that will satisfy and nourish you. Once you try the delish dishes in this cookbook, you and your air fryer are sure to become inseparable too.

It's important to think outside the box when it comes to trying out recipes in your air fryer. From roasted vegetables to empanadas, to baked eggs and vegan brownies, there's an option for everyone when you use your air fryer.

This cookbook is for people who want to create tasty dishes without spending all day in the kitchen. Most of the recipes can be prepared in 15 minutes or less. And most of them can be on the table in under an hour. With today's busy lifestyles, I know this is important to most of you.

In keeping with the latest health trends and diets, the recipes also include complete nutrition information. As a plus, there are recipes for those on a Vegan Diet as well as Mediterranean diet.

Let's delve in!

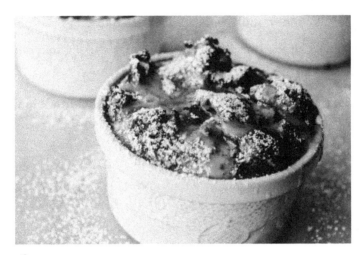

Serves: 3

INGREDIENTS

- 8 slices of bread
- ½ cup buttermilk
- ¼ cup honey
- 1 cup milk
- 2 eggs
- ½ tsp vanilla extract
- 2 tbsp butter, softened
- ¼ cup sugar
- 4 tbsp raisins
- 2 tbsp chopped hazelnuts
- Cinnamon for garnish

DIRECTIONS

1. Preheat the air fryer to 310 degrees F. Beat the eggs along with the buttermilk, honey, milk, vanilla, sugar, and butter. Stir in raisins and hazelnuts. Cut the bread into cubes and place them, in a bowl. Pour the milk mixture over the bread.

2. Let soak for 10 minutes. Cook the bread pudding for 30 minutes and garnish it with cinnamon.

Per serving: Calories: 529; Carbs: 77 g; Fat: 20 g; Protein: 13 g

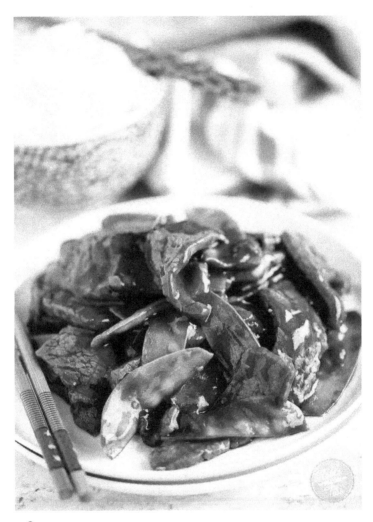

Serves: 2

Ingredients:

- 2 beef steaks, cut into strips

- Salt and black pepper to taste

- 14 ounces snow peas

- 2 tablespoons soy sauce

- 1 tablespoon olive oil

Directions:

1. Put all of the ingredients into a pan that fits your air fryer; toss well.

2. Place the pan in the fryer and cook at 390 degrees F for 25 minutes.

3. Divide everything between plates and serve.

Nutrition: calories 265, fat 11, fiber 4, carbs 22, protein 19

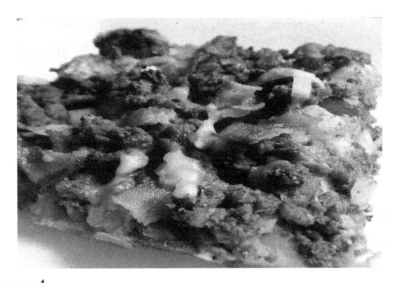

Serves: 4

Ingredients

- 1 lb ground beef

- ¼ teaspoon onion powder

- 4 eggs

- ½ cup heavy cream

- ¼ teaspoon ground pepper

- 1½ garlic cloves, crushed

- ½ lb bacon, cooked and chopped

- 3 oz. tomato paste

- ¼ teaspoon salt

- 6 oz. cheddar cheese, grated

Directions

1. Put the beef, bacon, garlic, and onion powder into the Air Fryer and 'sauté' for 5 minutes.
2. Combine the cream, eggs, salt, tomato paste, and cheddar cheese in a bowl.
3. Pour this mixture over the beef and bacon. Secure the lid.
4. Cook on 'the manual' function for 25 minutes at high pressure.
5. 'Natural release the steam for 5 minutes, then remove the lid.
6. Serve hot.

Nutrition Values (Per Serving): Calories: 823| Carbohydrate: 6.7g| Protein: 72.9g| Fat: 54.9g

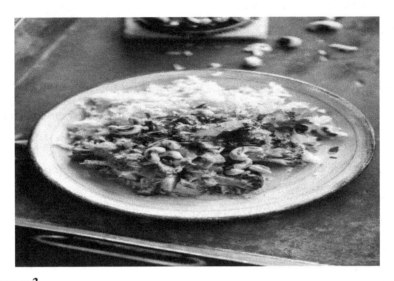

Serves: 3

Ingredients

- 1 lb cubed lamb stew meat

- 1 tablespoon fresh ginger, grated

- ½ teaspoon lime juice

- ¼ teaspoon black pepper

- ¾ cup diced tomatoes

- ½ teaspoon turmeric powder

- 1½ medium carrots, sliced

- 2 garlic cloves, minced

- ½ cup coconut milk

- ¼ teaspoon salt

- 1 tablespoon olive oil

- ½ medium onion, diced

- ½ medium zucchini, diced

Directions

1. Combine the garlic, ginger, salt, pepper, coconut milk, and lime juice in a bowl and add the meat to marinate for 30 minutes.

2. Put the oil and meat, along with the marinade, tomatoes, carrots, turmeric powder, and onions, into the Air Fryer.

3. Secure the lid and cook for 20 minutes on 'manual' function at high pressure.

4. 'Natural release' for 15 minutes, then remove the lid.

5. Add the zucchini to the curry and let it simmer for 5 minutes.

6. Serve hot.

Nutrition Values (Per Serving): Calories: 255 | Carbohydrate: 12.7g | Protein: 9,5g | Fat: 19.6g

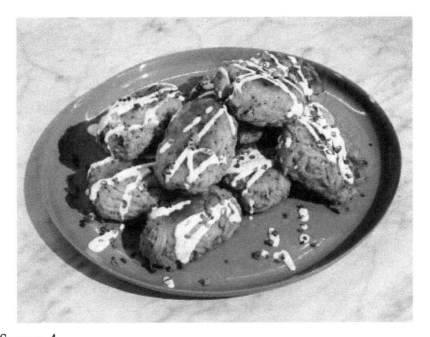

Serves: 4

Ingredients

- ¾ lbs lean ground beef

- 16 oz. frozen potato rounds, tater tots

- ¼ onion, chopped

- 8 oz. cream of chicken soup

- 2 tablespoons olive oil

Directions

1. Heat the oil in the Air Fryer on 'sauté' mode.

2. Stir in the beef and onion. Sauté for 5 minutes.

3. Add the cream of chicken soup and place the potato tater tots on top.

4. Secure the lid and cook for 25 minutes at medium pressure on the manual setting.

5. 'Natural release' for 5 minutes, then remove the lid.

6. Serve warm.

Nutrition Values (Per Serving): Calories: 1100| Carbohydrate: 92.7g| Protein: 35.2g| Fat: 63.4g| Sugar: 0.6g| Sodium: 1052mg

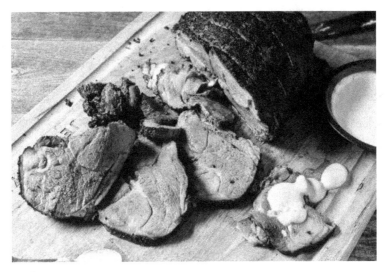

Serves: 6

Ingredients

- 2 lbs leg of lamb

- 1 teaspoon fine sea salt

- 2½ tablespoons olive oil

- 6 sprigs thyme

- 1½ cups bone broth

- 6 garlic cloves, minced

- 1½ teaspoons black pepper

- 1½ small onions

- ¾ cup orange juice

Directions

1. Add the salt, pepper, and garlic to the lamb and marinate.

2. Heat the oil in the Air Fryer using the 'sauté' function, then add the onions.

3. Cook for 4 minutes then remove the onions from the pot.

4. Put the marinated lamb in the pot and cook for 3 minutes on each side.

5. Stir in the broth, onions, orange juice, and thyme. Secure the lid.

6. Select 'meat stew' mode and cook for 40 minutes.

7. 'Natural release' the steam for 10 minutes, then remove the lid.

8. Serve hot.

Nutrition Values (Per Serving): Calories: 380| Carbohydrate: 6.3g| Protein: 48.1g| Fat: 17g

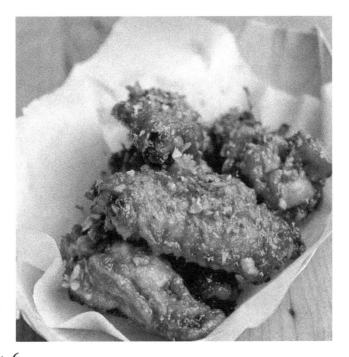

Serves: 6

Ingredients:

- 18 chicken wings; halved

- 1 tbsp. turmeric powder

- 1 tbsp. cumin; ground

- 2 tbsp. olive oil

- 1 tbsp. ginger; grated

- 1 tbsp. coriander; ground

- 1 tbsp. sweet paprika

- Salt and black pepper to the taste For the mint sauce:

- 3/4 cup cilantro

- Juice from 1/2 lime

- 1 cup mint leaves

- 1 small ginger piece; chopped

- 1 tbsp. olive oil

- 1 Serrano pepper; chopped

- 1 tbsp. water

- Salt and black pepper to the taste

Directions:

1. In a bowl, mix 1 tbsp. ginger with cumin, coriander, paprika, turmeric, salt, pepper, cayenne, and 2 tbsp. oil and stir well.

2. Add chicken wings pieces to this mix; toss to coat well and keep in the fridge for 10 minutes.

3. Transfer chicken to your air fryer's basket and cook at 370 °F, for 16 minutes; flipping them halfway.

4. In your blender, mix mint with cilantro, 1 small ginger piece, juice from 1/2 lime, 1 tbsp. olive oil, salt, pepper, water, and Serrano pepper and blend very well. Divide chicken wings on plates, drizzle the mint sauce all over, and serve.

Nutrition Facts (Per Serving): Calories: 300; Fat: 15; Fiber: 11; Carbs: 27; Protein: 16

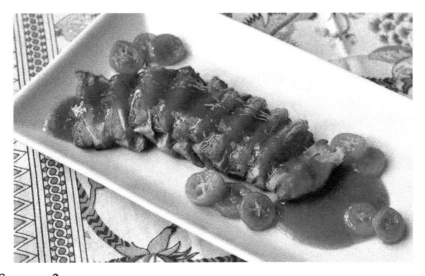

Serves: 2

Ingredients:

- 1 smoked duck breast; halved

- 1 tsp. honey

- 1 tsp. tomato paste

- 1 tbsp. mustard

- 1/2 tsp. apple vinegar

Directions:

1. In a bowl, mix honey with tomato paste, mustard, and vinegar, whisk well, add duck breast pieces, toss to coat well, transfer to your air fryer and cook at 370 °F, for 15 minutes.

2. Take duck breast out of the fryer, add to the honey mix, toss again, return to air fryer and cook at 370 °F, for 6 minutes more. Divide among plates and serve with a side salad.

Nutrition Facts (Per Serving): Calories: 274; Fat: 11; Fiber: 13; Carbs: 22; Protein: 13

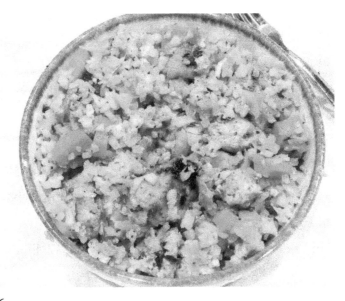

Serves: 6

Ingredients:

- 3 lbs. chicken thighs; boneless and skinless

- 3 bacon slices; chopped

- 3 carrots; chopped

- 2 bay leaves

- 1/4 cup red wine vinegar

- 4 garlic cloves; minced

- 4 tbsp. olive oil

- 1 tbsp. garlic powder

- 1 tbsp. Italian seasoning

- 24 oz. cauliflower rice

- 1 tsp. turmeric powder

- 1 cup beef stock

- Salt and black pepper to the taste

Directions:

1. Heat a pan that fits your air fryer over medium-high heat, add bacon, carrots, onion, and garlic; stir and cook for 8 minutes. 2. Add chicken, oil, vinegar, turmeric, garlic powder, Italian seasoning, and bay leaves; stir, introduce in your air fryer and cook at 360 °F, for 12 minutes. Add cauliflower rice and stock; stir, cook for 6 minutes more, divide among plates, and serve.

Nutrition Facts (Per Serving): Calories: 340; Fat: 12; Fiber: 12; Carbs: 16; Protein: 8

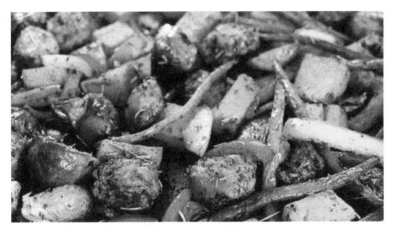

Serves: 4

Ingredients:

- 1/2 tsp. rosemary; dried

- 1/2 tsp. sage; dried

- 1/2 tsp. thyme; dried

- 1 yellow onion; chopped

- 1 carrot; chopped

- 3 garlic cloves; minced

- 2 lbs. turkey quarters

- 1 celery stalk; chopped

- 1 cup chicken stock

- 2 tbsp. olive oil

- 2 bay leaves

- Salt and black pepper to the taste

Directions:

1. Rub turkey quarters with salt, pepper, half of the oil, thyme, sage, rosemary, and thyme, put in your air fryer, and cook at 360 °F, for 20 minutes.

2. In a pan that fits your air fryer, mix the onion with carrot, garlic, celery, the rest of the oil, stock, bay leaves, salt, and pepper, and toss.

3. Add turkey, introduce everything in your air fryer and cook at 360 °F, for 14 minutes more. Divide everything between plates and serve.

Nutrition Facts (Per Serving): Calories: 362; Fat: 12; Fiber: 16; Carbs: 22; Protein: 17

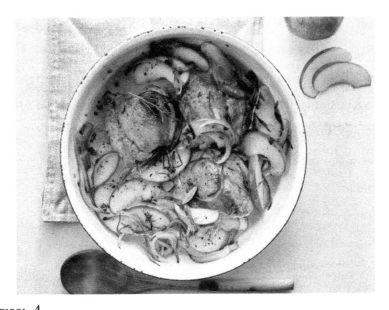

Serves: 4

Ingredients:

- 8 chicken thighs; bone-in and skin on

- 1 tbsp. apple cider vinegar

- 3 tbsp. onion; chopped

- 1 tbsp. ginger; grated

- 1/2 tsp. thyme; dried

- 3 apples; cored and cut into quarters

- 3/4 cup apple juice

- 1/2 cup maple syrup

- Salt and black pepper to the taste

Directions:

1. In a bowl, mix chicken with salt, pepper, vinegar, onion, ginger, thyme, apple juice, and maple syrup; toss well, cover, and keep in the fridge for 12 hours.
2. Transfer this whole mix to a baking dish that fits your air fryer, add apple pieces, place in your air fryer and cook at 350 °F, for 30 minutes. Divide among plates and serve warm.

Nutrition Facts (Per Serving): Calories: 314; Fat: 8; Fiber: 11; Carbs: 34; Protein: 22

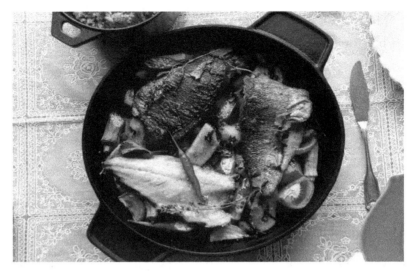

Serves: 2

Ingredients: For the fish

- 2 medium cod fillets

- 2 tbsp coconut milk

- Salt and pepper to taste

  For the sauce

- 1/2 cup coconut milk

- 1/2 cup chicken broth

- 1/2 tsp white sugar 1 tsp lime juice

- 2 slices ginger root

- Chopped cilantro for serving

Directions:

1. Preheat the water bath to 135 degrees F.

2. Rub the sea bass fillets with salt, pepper, and coconut milk and put them into the vacuum bag.

3. Seal the bag and set the timer for 30 minutes.

4. While the fish is cooking, make the sauce.

5. Combine the chicken broth and coconut milk in a pan, and simmer for about 10 minutes over medium heat.

6. Add the lime juice, sugar and ginger root, mix well and take the sauce off the heat. Close the pan with the lid and set it aside for a couple of minutes.

7. Put the fish in bowls, pour the sauce over and serve topped with the freshly chopped cilantro.

Nutrition per serving: Calories: 580, Protein: 22 g, Fats: 15 g, Carbs: 88 g

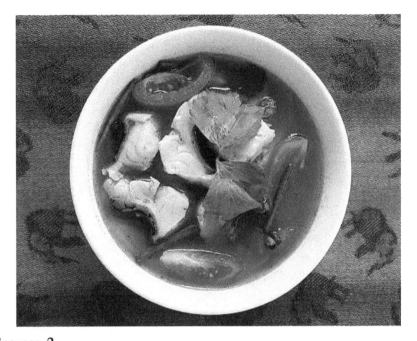

Serves: 2

Ingredients:

- 2 medium fish fillets (any white fish of your choice)
- 2 tbsp Tom Yum paste
- Fresh cilantro for serving
- 1 tbsp lime juice for serving

Directions:

1. Preheat the water bath to 135 degrees F.
2. Rub the fillets with the Tom Yum paste, and put them into the vacuum bag.
3. Seal the bag and set the timer for 30 minutes.

4. Serve over white rice sprinkled with lime juice and topped with freshly chopped cilantro.

Nutrition per serving: Calories: 200, Protein: 20 g, Fats: 5 g, Carbs: 14 g

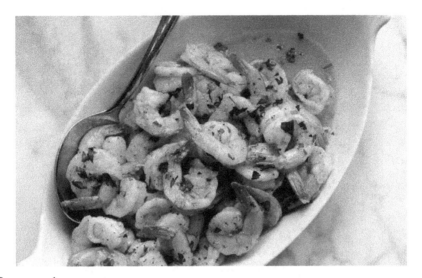

Serves: 4

Ingredients:

- 16 shrimps, peeled and deveined
- 1 shallot, minced
- 1 tbsp unsalted butter, melted
- 2 tsp thyme
- 1 tsp lemon zest, grated

Directions:

1. Preheat your cooking machine to 125 degrees F.
2. Put all ingredients in the vacuum bag.
3. Seal the bag, put it into the water bath and set the timer for 25 minutes.
4. Serve immediately as an appetizer or tossed with penne pasta.

Nutrition per serving: Calories: Protein: g, Fats: g, Carbs: g

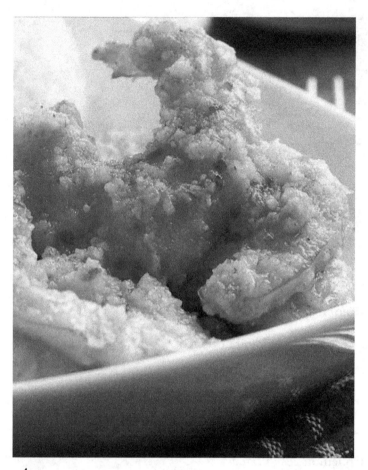

Serves: 4

Ingredients:

- 16 shrimps, peeled and deveined
- 1 shallot, minced
- 1 tbsp unsalted butter, melted
- 2 garlic cloves, minced

Directions:

1. Preheat your cooking machine to 125 degrees F.

2. Put all ingredients in the vacuum bag.

3. Seal the bag, put it into the water bath and set the timer for 25 minutes.

4. Serve immediately as an appetizer or tossed with penne pasta.

Nutrition per serving: Calories: 202, Protein: 27 g, Fats: 1 g, Carbs: 9 g

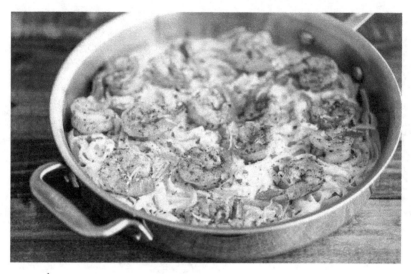

Serves: 4

Ingredients:

- 16 shrimps, peeled and deveined
- 1 shallot, minced
- 1 tbsp unsalted butter, melted
- 1 tbsp Cajun seasoning
- 2 garlic cloves, minced
- 1 tbsp lemon juice
- Freshly ground black pepper to taste
- 4 tbsp freshly chopped parsley

Directions:

1. Preheat your cooking machine to 125 degrees F.
2. Put all ingredients except parsley into the vacuum bag.

3. Seal the bag, put it into the water bath and set the timer for 25 minutes.
4. Serve immediately as an appetizer garnished with the chopped parsley.

Nutrition per serving: Calories: 133, Protein: 18 g, Fats: 7 g, Carbs: 1 g

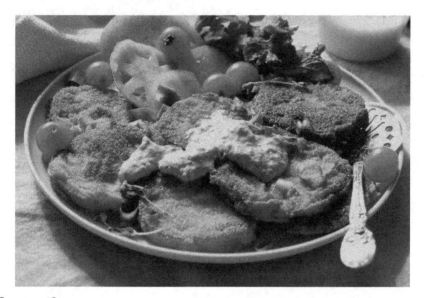

Serves: 8

Ingredients:

- 1 jalapeno pepper; chopped

- 4 garlic cloves; minced

- 1/2 tsp. oregano; dried

- 1/4 cup basil; chopped.

- 2 lbs. cherry tomatoes; halved

- Salt and black pepper to the taste

- 1/4 cup olive oil

- 1/2 cup parmesan; grated

Directions:

1. In a bowl; mix tomatoes with garlic, jalapeno, season with salt, pepper, and oregano and drizzle the oil, toss to coat, introduce in your air fryer and cook at 380 °F, for 15 minutes

2. Transfer tomatoes to a bowl, add basil and parmesan, toss and serve.

Nutrition Facts (Per Serving): Calories: 140; Fat: 2; Fiber: 2; Carbs:6; Protein: 8

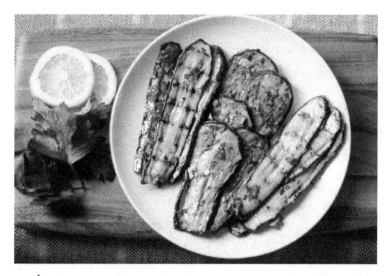

Serves: 4

Ingredients:

- 1 eggplant; roughly cubed

- 3 zucchinis; roughly cubed

- 2 tbsp. lemon juice

- 1 tsp. thyme; dried

- Salt and black pepper to the taste

- 1 tsp. oregano; dried

- 3 tbsp. olive oil

Directions:

1. Put eggplant in a dish that fits your air fryer, add zucchinis, lemon juice, salt, pepper, thyme, oregano and olive oil, toss, introduce in your air fryer and cook at 360 °F, for 8 minutes

2. 2. Divide among plates and serve right away.

Nutrition Facts (Per Serving): Calories: 152; Fat: 5; Fiber: 7; Carbs:19; Protein: 5

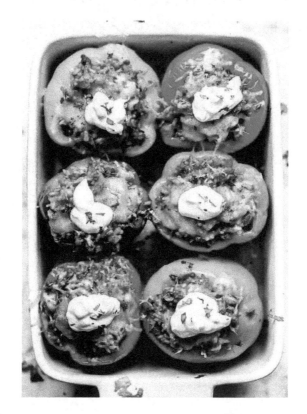

Serves: 4

Ingredients:

- 4 bell peppers; tops cut off and seeds removed

- 1/2 cup tomato juice

- 1/4 cup yellow onion; chopped

- 1/4 cup green peppers; chopped.

- 2 cups tomato sauce

- 2 tbsp. jarred jalapenos; chopped.

- 4 chicken breasts

- 1 cup tomatoes; chopped

- Salt and black pepper to the taste

- 2 tsp. onion powder

- 1/2 tsp. red pepper; crushed

- 1 tsp. chili powder

- 1/2 tsp. garlic powder

- 1 tsp. cumin; ground

Directions:

1.   In a pan that fits your air fryer, mix chicken breasts with tomato juice, jalapenos, tomatoes, onion, green peppers, salt, pepper, onion powder, red pepper, chili powder, garlic powder, oregano and cumin; stir well, introduce in your air fryer and cook at 350 °F, for 15 minutes

2.   Shred meat using 2 forks; stir, stuff bell peppers with this mix, place them in your air fryer and cook at 320 °F, for 10 minutes more.

3.   Divide stuffed peppers between plates and serve

Nutrition Facts (Per Serving): Calories: 180; Fat: 4; Fiber: 3; Carbs:7; Protein: 14

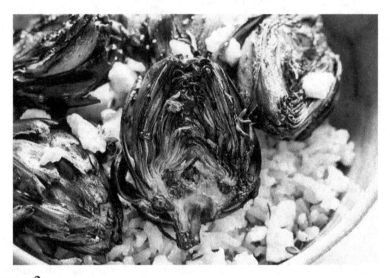

Serves: 2

Ingredients:

- 4 big artichokes; trimmed

- 2 tbsp. lemon juice

- 2 tsp. balsamic vinegar

- 1 tsp. oregano; dried

- 1/4 cup extra virgin olive oil

- 2 garlic cloves; minced

- Salt and black pepper to the taste

Directions:

1.   Season artichokes with salt and pepper, rub them with half of the oil and half of the lemon juice, put them in your air fryer and cook at

2.   360 °F, for 7 minutes

3.   . Meanwhile; in a bowl, mix the rest of the lemon juice with vinegar, the remaining oil, salt, pepper, garlic, and oregano and stir very well 3. Arrange artichokes on a platter, drizzle the balsamic vinaigrette over them and serve.

Nutrition Facts (Per Serving): Calories: 200; Fat: 3; Fiber: 6; Carbs:12; Protein: 4

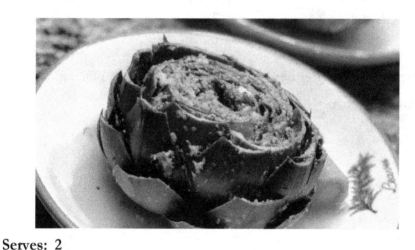

Serves: 2

Ingredients:

- 2 artichokes; trimmed
- 2 garlic cloves; minced
- A drizzle of olive oil • 1 tbsp. lemon juice For the sauce:
- 3 anchovy fillets
- 1/4 cup coconut oil
- 1/4 cup extra virgin olive oil
- 3 garlic cloves

Directions:

1. In a bowl; mix artichokes with oil, 2 garlic cloves and lemon juice, toss well, transfer to your air fryer, cook at 350 °F, for 6 minutes and divide among plates

2. In your food processor, mix coconut oil with anchovy, 3 garlic cloves, and olive oil, blend very well, drizzle over artichokes and serve.

Nutrition Facts (Per Serving): Calories: 261; Fat: 4; Fiber: 7; Carbs:20; Protein: 12

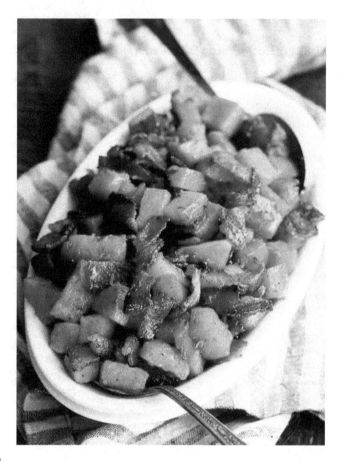

Serve 4:

Ingredients:

- 1 large butternut squash, peeled, halved, seeded, and cut into 1-inch chunks

- 1 teaspoon extra-virgin olive oil or canola oil

- 2 tablespoons maple syrup

- 1 teaspoon ground cinnamon

- 1/2 teaspoon ground cardamom
- 1/2 teaspoon dried thyme
- 1/2 teaspoon sea salt

Directions:

1. Preheat the air fryer to 390°F. Place the squash into a large mixing bowl. Add the oil, maple syrup, cinnamon, cardamom, thyme, and salt, and toss to coat the squash.

2. Transfer the squash to the air fryer basket. Cook for 20 minutes or until browned, shaking halfway through the cooking time.

   Serves: 4

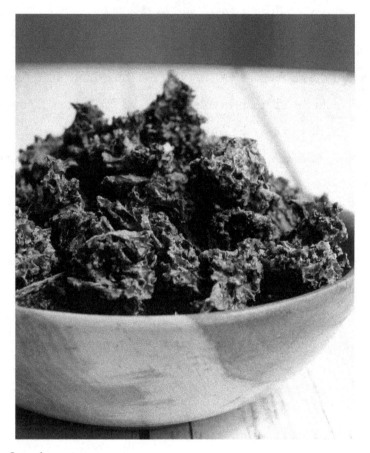

Serve 2 to 4:

Ingredients:

- 8 cups stemmed kale
- 1 teaspoon canola oil or extra-virgin olive oil
- 1 teaspoon rice vinegar
- 1 teaspoon soy sauce
- 2 tablespoons nutritional yeast

Directions:

1. Wash and drain the kale. Transfer it to a large bowl. Tear the kale into 2-inch pieces. Avoid tearing pieces too small, as some air fryers, with powerful forced air, may pull the kale into the heating element.

2. Add the oil, vinegar, soy sauce, and nutritional yeast to the bowl. Using your hands, massage all the ingredients into the kale for about 2 minutes.

3. Transfer the kale to the air fryer basket. Cook at 360°F for 5 minutes. Shake the basket. Increase the heat to 390°F and cook for 5 to 7 more minutes.

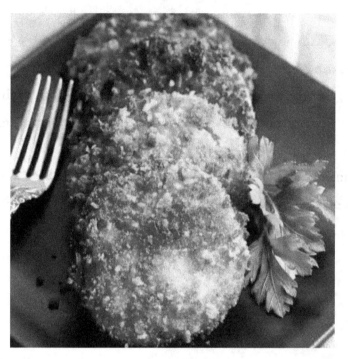

Serve 6 to 8:

Ingredients:

- 1/2 cup potato starch
- 1 cup soy flour, divided
- 1/4 cup soymilk
- 2 tablespoons nutritional yeast
- 1/2 to 1 teaspoon hot sauce
- 1/4 cup almond flour
- 1/4 cup panko bread crumbs
- 1 teaspoon smoked paprika

- 1 teaspoon sea salt

- 1/4 teaspoon black pepper

- 2 large green or heirloom tomatoes, cut into 1/2-inch thick slices

- 2 to 4 spritzes canola oil

Directions:

1. In a shallow dish, combine the potato starch and 1/2 cup of soy flour.

2. In a second shallow dish, combine the milk, nutritional yeast, and hot sauce.

3. In a third shallow dish, combine the remaining 1/2 cup soy flour, almond flour, panko bread crumbs, smoked paprika, salt, and pepper.

4. Coat the tomatoes in the potato starch mixture. Shake off any excess starch and then dip the tomatoes in the milk mixture to coat. Shake off any excess milk and then dredge the tomatoes in the seasoned soy flour mixture.

5. Spritz the air fryer basket with the oil. Place as many tomatoes on the air fryer basket as you can. Spritz the top of the tomatoes with more oil.

6. Cook at 320°F for 3 minutes. Shake the air fryer basket gently. Increase the heat to 400°F and cook for 2 more minutes.

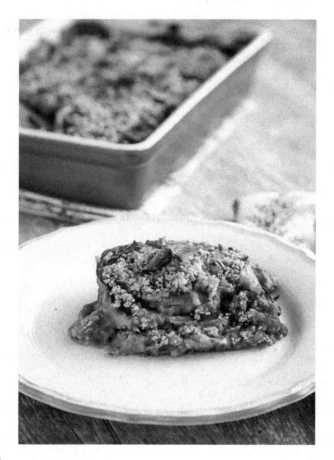

Serve 4:

Ingredients:

- 1 medium eggplant
- 1/2 cup unbleached all-purpose flour
- 1 Flax Egg (see here) or equivalent Follow Your Heart Vegan Egg or Ener-G Egg Replacer
- 1 1/2 cups panko bread crumbs

- 2 to 4 spritzes extra-virgin olive oil
- 1/2 cup marinara sauce
- 1/2 cup shredded nondairy Parmesan cheese

Directions:

1. Wash the eggplant and pat dry. Slice the eggplant, making 8 (1/2-inch thick) rounds.

2. Set up a three-part dredging station using three shallow bowls, with the flour in the first, flax egg in the second, and panko bread crumbs in the third. Spritz the air fryer basket with the oil.

3. Dredge an eggplant round into the flour, coating well. Dip the eggplant rounds into the flax egg, and then dredge it in the panko bread crumbs. Shake off any excess bread crumbs and place the eggplant rounds into the air fryer basket. Repeat this process with more of the eggplant rounds. If you have a rack accessory, place it in the air fryer basket and continue coating the remaining eggplant rounds and place them on the rack. If you have a smaller air fryer or no rack to add a second level of cooking, air-fry the eggplant rounds in 2 or 3 batches. Spritz the top of each eggplant round with olive oil. Cook at 360°F for 12 minutes, until golden brown.

4. Heat the marinara sauce in a small saucepan over medium heat.

5. After 12 minutes, open the air fryer and add 1 tablespoon cheese to each eggplant round and cook for 2 minutes longer. To serve, plate 3 eggplant rounds per person on a small plate. Spoon 2 tablespoons of marinara sauce over the eggplant.

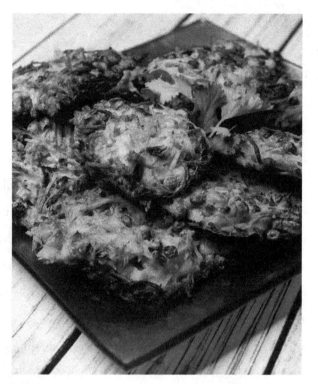

Serve 10 to 12:

Ingredients:

- 3 tablespoons ground flaxseed

- 1/2 cup water

- 2 medium russet potatoes

- 2 cups frozen mixed vegetables (carrots, peas, and corn), thawed and drained

- 1 cup frozen peas, thawed and drained

- 1/2 cup coarsely chopped onion

- 1/4 cup finely chopped fresh cilantro

- 1/2 cup unbleached all-purpose flour

- 1/2 teaspoon sea salt

- Extra-virgin olive oil for spritzing

Directions:

1. In a small bowl, make a flax egg by mixing the flaxseed and water with a fork or small whisk.

2. Peel the potatoes and shred them into a bowl. (Or use the grater blade in a food processor; if doing so, transfer the shredded potatoes back into a bowl.) Add the mixed vegetables and onion to the potatoes. Add the cilantro and flax egg and stir to combine. Add the flour and salt and combine well. Preheat the air fryer to 360°F for 3 minutes.

3. Scoop out 1/3 cup of the potato mixture to form a patty. Repeat this process until all of the mixtures is used to make fritter patties.

4. Spritz the fritters with the oil. Transfer the fritters to the air fryer basket (you may need to do several batches, depending upon the size of your air fryer). Cook the fritters for 15 minutes, flipping halfway through the cooking time.

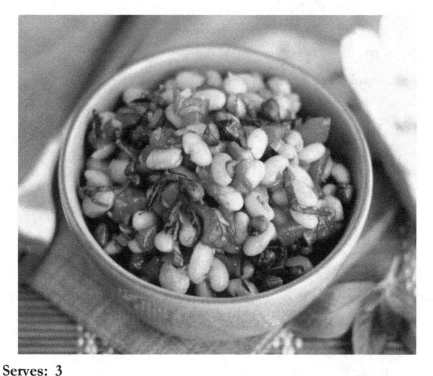

Serves: 3

Ingredients:

- Olive oil cooking spray
- 2 (15-ounce) cans of white beans, or cannellini beans, drained and rinsed
- 1 red bell pepper, diced
- ½ red onion, diced
- 3 garlic cloves, minced
- 1 tablespoon olive oil
- ¼ to ½ teaspoon salt
- ½ teaspoon black pepper

- 1 rosemary sprig
- 1 bay leaf

Directions:

1. . Preheat the air fryer to 360°F. Lightly coat the inside of a 5-cup capacity casserole dish with olive oil cooking spray. (The shape of the casserole dish will depend upon the size of the air fryer, but it needs to be able to hold at least 5 cups.)

2. . In a large bowl, combine the beans, bell pepper, onion, garlic, olive oil, salt, and pepper.

3. . Pour the bean mixture into the prepared casserole dish, place the rosemary and bay leaf on top, and then place the casserole dish into the air fryer.

4. . Roast for 15 minutes.

5. . Remove the rosemary and bay leaves, then stir well before serving.

PER SERVING: Calories: 196; Total Fat: 5g; Saturated Fat: 0g; Protein: 10g; Total Carbohydrates: 30g; Fiber: 1g; Sugar: 2g; Cholesterol: 0mg

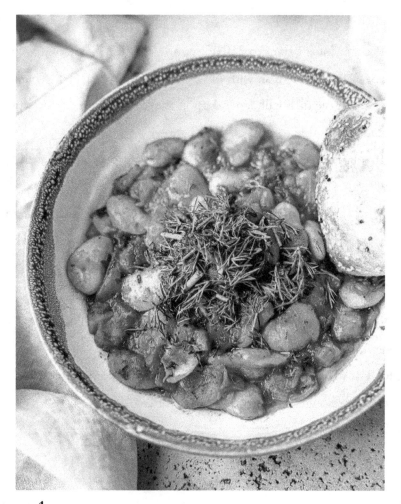

Serves: 1

Ingredients:

- 1 (15-ounce) can cannellini beans, drained and rinsed

- 1 (15-ounce) can great northern beans, drained and rinsed

- ½ yellow onion, diced

- 1 (8-ounce) can tomato sauce

- 1½ tablespoons raw honey
- ¼ cup olive oil
- 2 garlic cloves, minced
- 2 tablespoons chopped fresh dill
- ½ teaspoon salt
- ½ teaspoon black pepper
- 1 bay leaf
- 1 tablespoon balsamic vinegar
- 2 ounces feta cheese, crumbled, for serving

Directions:

1. . Preheat the air fryer to 360°F. Lightly coat the inside of a 5-cup capacity casserole dish with olive oil cooking spray. (The shape of the casserole dish will depend upon the size of the air fryer, but it needs to be able to hold at least 5 cups.)

2. . In a large bowl, combine all ingredients except the feta cheese and stir until well combined.

3. . Pour the bean mixture into the prepared casserole dish.

4. . Bake in the air fryer for 30 minutes.

5. . Remove from the air fryer and remove and discard the bay leaf. Sprinkle crumbled feta over the top before serving.

PER SERVING: Calories: 397; Total Fat: 18g; Saturated Fat: 4g; Protein: 14g; Total Carbohydrates: 48g; Fiber: 16g; Sugar: 11g; Cholesterol: 13mg

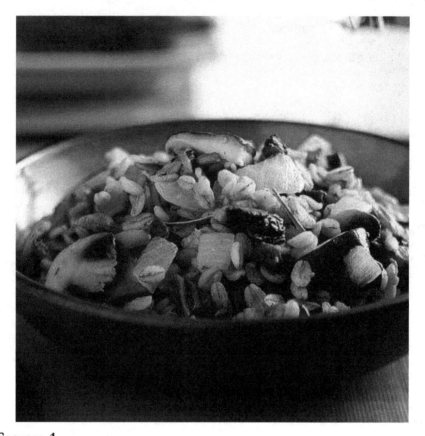

Serves: 1

Ingredients:

- Olive oil cooking spray
- 2 tablespoons olive oil
- 8 ounces button mushrooms, diced
- ½ yellow onion, diced
- 2 garlic cloves, minced
- 1 cup pearl barley

- 2 cups vegetable broth
- 1 tablespoon fresh thyme, chopped
- ½ teaspoon salt
- ¼ teaspoon smoked paprika
- Fresh parsley, for garnish

Directions:

1. . Preheat the air fryer to 380°F. Lightly coat the inside of a 5-cup capacity casserole dish with olive oil cooking spray. (The shape of the casserole dish will depend upon the size of the air fryer, but it needs to be able to hold at least 5 cups.)

2. . In a large skillet, heat the olive oil over medium heat. Add the mushrooms and onion and cook, stirring occasionally, for 5 minutes, or until the mushrooms begin to brown.

3. . Add the garlic and cook for an additional 2 minutes. Transfer the vegetables to a large bowl.

4. . Add the barley, broth, thyme, salt, and paprika.

5. . Pour the barley-and-vegetable mixture into the prepared casserole dish, and place the dish into the air fryer. Bake for 15 minutes.

6. . Stir the barley mixture. Reduce the heat to 360°F, then return the barley to the air fryer and bake for 15 minutes more.

7. . Remove from the air fryer and let sit for 5 minutes before fluffing with a fork and topping with fresh parsley.

PER SERVING: Calories: 263; Total Fat: 8g; Saturated Fat: 1g; Protein: 7g; Total Carbohydrates: 44g; Fiber: 9g; Sugar: 3g; Cholesterol: 0mg

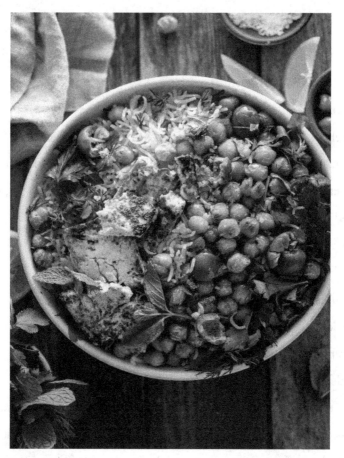

Serves: 4-6

Ingredients:

- Olive oil cooking spray

- 1 cup long-grain brown rice

- 2 ¼ cups chicken stock

- 1 (15.5-ounce) can chickpeas, drained and rinsed

- ½ cup diced carrot

- ½ cup green peas
- 1 teaspoon ground cumin
- ½ teaspoon ground turmeric
- ½ teaspoon ground ginger
- ½ teaspoon onion powder
- ½ teaspoon salt
- ¼ teaspoon ground cinnamon
- ¼ teaspoon garlic powder
- ¼ teaspoon black pepper
- Fresh parsley, for garnish

Directions:

1. . Preheat the air fryer to 380°F. Lightly coat the inside of a 5-cup capacity casserole dish with olive oil cooking spray. (The shape of the casserole dish will depend upon the size of the air fryer, but it needs to be able to hold at least 5 cups.)

2. . In the casserole dish, combine the rice, stock, chickpeas, carrot, peas, cumin, turmeric, ginger, onion powder, salt, cinnamon, garlic powder, and black pepper. Stir well to combine.

3. . Cover loosely with aluminum foil.

4. . Place the covered casserole dish into the air fryer and bake for 20 minutes. Remove from the air fryer and stir well.

5. .Place the casserole back into the air fryer, uncovered, and bake for 25 minutes more.

6. Fluff with a spoon and sprinkle with fresh chopped parsley before serving.

PER SERVING: Calories: 204; Total Fat: 2g; Saturated Fat: 0g; Protein: 7g; Total Carbohydrates: 40g; Fiber: 5g; Sugar: 4g; Cholesterol: 0mg

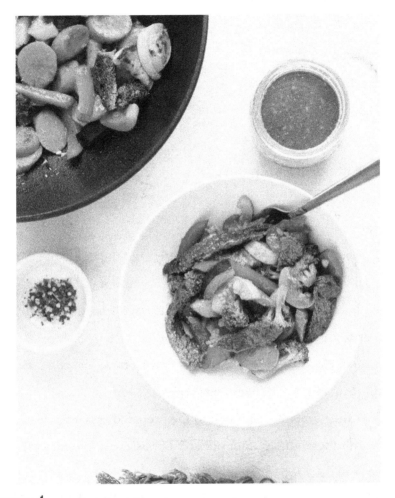

Serves: 4

Ingredients:

- Olive oil cooking spray

- 2 large potatoes, cubed

- 2 carrots, sliced

- 1 small rutabaga, cubed

- 2 celery stalks, chopped
- ½ teaspoon smoked paprika
- ¼ cup plus 1 tablespoon olive oil, divided
- 2 rosemary sprigs
- 1 cup buckwheat groats
- 2 cups vegetable broth
- 2 garlic cloves, minced
- ½ yellow onion, chopped
- 1 teaspoon salt

Directions:

1. . Preheat the air fryer to 380°F. Lightly coat the inside of a 5-cup capacity casserole dish with olive oil cooking spray. (The shape of the casserole dish will depend upon the size of the air fryer, but it needs to be able to hold at least 5 cups.)

2. . In a large bowl, toss the potatoes, carrots, rutabaga, and celery with the paprika and ¼ cup olive oil.

3. . Pour the vegetable mixture into the prepared casserole dish and top with the rosemary sprigs. Place the casserole dish into the air fryer and bake for 15 minutes.

4. . While the vegetables are cooking, rinse and drain the buckwheat groats.

5. . In a medium saucepan over medium-high heat, combine the groats, vegetable broth, garlic, onion, and salt with the remaining 1 tablespoon olive oil. Bring the mixture to a boil, then reduce the heat to low, cover, and cook for 10 to 12 minutes.

6. . Remove the casserole dish from the air fryer. Remove the rosemary sprigs and discard. Pour the cooked buckwheat into the dish with the vegetables and stir to combine. Cover with aluminum foil and bake for an additional 15 minutes.

7. . Stir before serving.

PER SERVING: Calories: 344; Total Fat: 13g; Saturated Fat: 2g; Protein: 8g; Total Carbohydrates: 50g; Fiber: 8g; Sugar: 4g; Cholesterol: 0mg

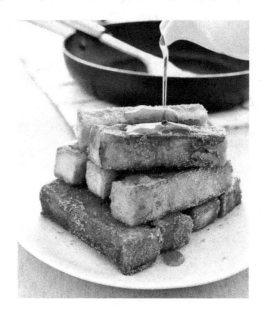

Serves: 6

Ingredients:

- 1½ teaspoons cinnamon

- 1½ teaspoons vanilla extract

- ½ cup sugar

- 2 teaspoons ground black pepper

- 2 tablespoons melted coconut oil

- 12 slices whole-wheat bread

Directions:

1. Combine all the ingredients, except for the bread, in a large bowl. Stir to mix well.

2. Dunk the bread in the bowl of mixture gently to coat and infuse well. Shake the excess off. Arrange the bread slices in the air fryer basket.

3. Put the air fryer basket on the baking pan and slide into Rack Position 2, select Air Fry, set temperature to 400°F (205°C), and set time to 5 minutes.

4. Flip the bread halfway through.

5. When cooking is complete, the bread should be golden brown.

6. Remove the bread slices from the oven and slice to serve.

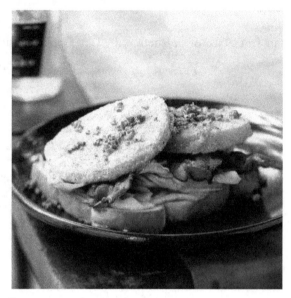

Serves: 12 slices

Ingredients:

- ½ cup all-purpose flour
- 1 egg
- ½ cup buttermilk
- 1 cup cornmeal
- 1 cup panko
- 2 green tomatoes, cut into ¼-inch-thick slices, patted dry
- ½ teaspoon salt
- ½ teaspoon ground black pepper
- Cooking spray

Directions:

1. Spritz a baking sheet with cooking spray.

2. Pour the flour into a bowl. Whisk the egg and buttermilk in a second bowl. Combine the cornmeal and panko in a third bowl.

3. Dredge the tomato slices in the bowl of flour first, then into the egg mixture, and then dunk the slices into the cornmeal mixture. Shake the excess off.

4. Transfer the well-coated tomato slices to the baking sheet and sprinkle with salt and ground black pepper. Spritz the tomato slices with cooking spray.

5. Put the air fryer basket on the baking pan and slide into Rack Position 2, select Air Fry, set temperature to 400°F (205°C), and set time to 8 minutes.

6. Flip the slices halfway through the cooking time.

7. When cooking is complete, the tomato slices should be crispy and lightly browned. Remove the baking sheet from the oven.

8. Serve immediately.

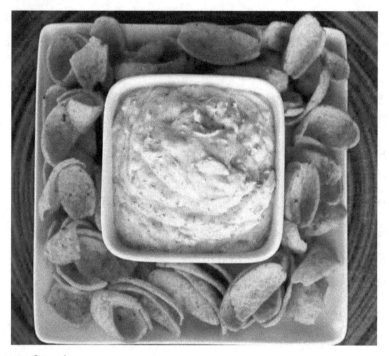

Serves: 2 to 4

Ingredients:

- 2 large russet potatoes, sliced into ⅛-inch slices, rinsed
- Sea salt and freshly ground black pepper, to taste
- Cooking spray
- Lemony Cream Dip:
- ½ cup sour cream
- ¼ teaspoon lemon juice
- 2 scallions, white part only, minced
- 1 tablespoon olive oil
- ¼ teaspoon salt

- Freshly ground black pepper, to taste

Directions:

1. Soak the potato slices in water for 10 minutes, then pat dry with paper towels.
2. Transfer the potato slices to the air fryer basket. Spritz the slices with cooking spray.
3. Put the air fryer basket on the baking pan and slide into Rack Position 2, select Air Fry, set temperature to 300°F (150°C), and set time to 15 minutes.
4. Stir the potato slices three times during cooking. Sprinkle with salt and ground black pepper at the last minute.
5. Meanwhile, combine the ingredients for the dip in a small bowl. Stir to mix well.
6. When cooking is complete, the potato slices will be crispy and golden brown. Remove from the oven and serve the potato chips immediately with the dip.

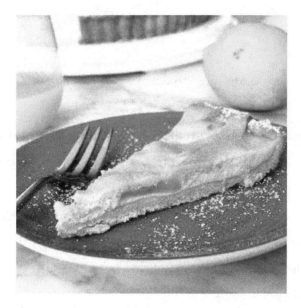

Serves: 4

Ingredients:

- 2 large Bartlett pears, peeled, cut in half, cored
- 3 tablespoons melted butter
- ½ teaspoon ground ginger
- ¼ teaspoon ground cardamom
- 3 tablespoons brown sugar
- ½ cup whole-milk ricotta cheese
- 1 teaspoon pure lemon extract
- 1 teaspoon pure almond extract
- 1 tablespoon honey, plus additional for drizzling

Directions:

1. Toss the pears with butter, ginger, cardamom, and sugar in a large bowl. Toss to coat well. Arrange the pears in the baking pan, cut side down.

2. Put the air fryer basket on the baking pan and slide into Rack Position 2, select Air Fry, set temperature to 375°F (190°C), and set time to 8 minutes.

3. After 5 minutes, remove the pan and flip the pears. Return to the oven and continue cooking.

4. When cooking is complete, the pears should be soft and browned. Remove from the oven.

5. In the meantime, combine the remaining ingredients in a separate bowl. Whip for 1 minute with a hand mixer until the mixture is puffed.

6. Divide the mixture into four bowls, then put the pears over the mixture and drizzle with more honey to serve.

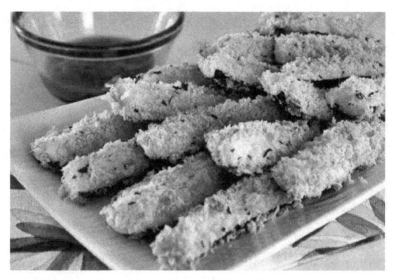

Serves: 4

Ingredients:

- 1 medium zucchini, cut into 48 sticks
- ¼ cup seasoned bread crumbs
- 1 tablespoon melted buttery spread
- Cooking spray

Directions:

1. Spritz the air fryer basket with cooking spray and set it aside.

2. In 2 different shallow bowls, add the seasoned bread crumbs and the buttery spread.

3. One by one, dredge the zucchini sticks into the buttery spread, then roll in the bread crumbs to coat evenly. Arrange the crusted sticks in the basket.

4. Put the air fryer basket on the baking pan and slide into Rack Position 2, select Air Fry, set temperature to 360°F (182°C), and set time to 10 minutes.

5. Stir the sticks halfway through the cooking time.

6. When done, the sticks should be golden brown and crispy. Transfer the fries to a plate. Rest for 5 minutes and serve warm.

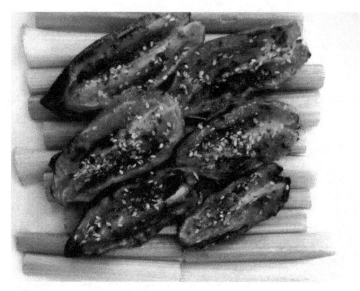

Serves: 4 to 6

Ingredients:

- 2 pounds (907 g) cherry tomatoes
- 2 tablespoons olive oil
- 2 teaspoons balsamic vinegar
- ½ teaspoon salt
- ½ teaspoon ground black pepper

Directions:

1. Toss the cherry tomatoes with olive oil in a large bowl to coat well. Pour the tomatoes into the baking pan.

2. Put the air fryer basket on the baking pan and slide into Rack Position 2, select Air Fry, set temperature to 400°F (205°C), and set time to 10 minutes.

3. Stir the tomatoes halfway through the cooking time.

4. When cooking is complete, the tomatoes will be blistered and lightly wilted.

5. Transfer the blistered tomatoes to a large bowl and toss with balsamic vinegar, salt, and black pepper before serving.

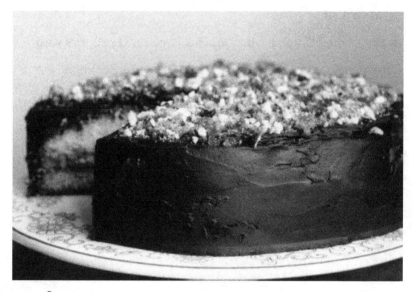

Serves: 8

Ingredients:

- 1 cup all-purpose flour
- ⅔ cup granulated white sugar
- ¼ cup unsweetened cocoa powder
- ¾ teaspoon baking soda
- ¼ teaspoon salt
- ⅔ cup buttermilk
- 2 tablespoons plus 2 teaspoons vegetable oil
- 1 teaspoon vanilla extract
- Cooking spray

Directions:

1. Spritz the baking pan with cooking spray.

2. Combine the flour, cocoa powder, baking soda, sugar, and salt in a large bowl. Stir to mix well.

3. Mix in the buttermilk, vanilla, and vegetable oil. Keep stirring until it forms a grainy and thick dough.

4. Scrape the chocolate batter from the bowl and transfer to the pan, level the batter in an even layer with a spatula.

5. Slide the baking pan into Rack Position 1, select Convection Bake set the temperature to 325°F (163°C), and set time to 20 minutes.

6. After 15 minutes, remove the pan from the oven. Check the doneness. Return the pan to the oven and continue cooking.

7. When done, a toothpick inserted in the center should come out clean.

8. Invert the cake on a cooling rack and allow it to cool for 15 minutes before slicing to serve.

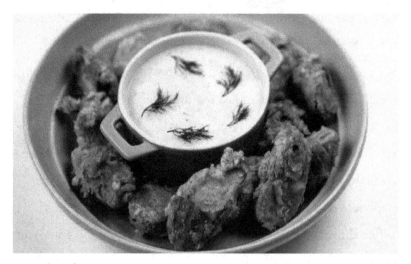

Serves: 6 to 8

Ingredients:

Buttermilk Dressing:

- ¼ cup buttermilk
- ¼ cup chopped scallions
- ¾ cup mayonnaise
- ½ cup sour cream
- ½ teaspoon cayenne pepper
- ½ teaspoon onion powder
- ½ teaspoon garlic powder
- 1 tablespoon chopped chives
- 2 tablespoons chopped fresh dill
- Kosher salt and ground black pepper, to taste

Fried Dill Pickles:

- ¾ cup all-purpose flour
- 1 (2-pound / 907-g) jar kosher dill pickles, cut into 4 spears, drained
- 2½ cups panko bread crumbs
- 2 eggs, beaten with 2 tablespoons water
- Kosher salt and ground black pepper, to taste
- Cooking spray

Directions:

1. Combine the ingredients for the dressing in a bowl. Stir to mix well.
2. Wrap the bowl in plastic and refrigerate for 30 minutes or until ready to serve.
3. Pour the flour into a bowl and sprinkle with salt and ground black pepper. Stir to mix well. Put the bread crumbs in a separate bowl. Pour the beaten eggs into a third bowl.
4. Dredge the pickle spears in the flour, then into the eggs, and then into the panko to coat well. Shake the excess off.
5. Arrange the pickle spears in a single layer in the air fryer basket and spritz with cooking spray.
6. Put the air fryer basket on the baking pan and slide into Rack Position 2, select Air Fry, set temperature to 400°F (205°C), and set time to 8 minutes.
7. Flip the pickle spears halfway through the cooking time.
8. When cooking is complete, remove it from the oven.
9. Serve the pickle spears with buttermilk dressing.

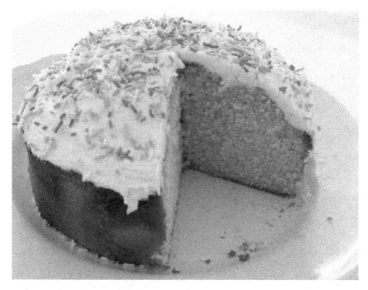

Serves: 8

Ingredients:

- 1 cup all-purpose flour

- 1¼ teaspoons baking powder

- ¼ teaspoon salt

- ½ cup plus 1½ tablespoons granulated white sugar

- 9½ tablespoons butter, at room temperature

- 2 large eggs

- 1 large egg yolk

- 2½ tablespoons milk

- 1 teaspoon vanilla extract

- Cooking spray

Directions:

1. Spritz the baking pan with cooking spray.
2. Combine the flour, baking powder, and salt in a large bowl. Stir to mix well.
3. Whip the sugar and butter in a separate bowl with a hand mixer on medium speed for 3 minutes.
4. Whip the eggs, egg yolk, milk, and vanilla extract into the sugar and butter mix with a hand mixer.
5. Pour in the flour mixture and whip with a hand mixer until sanity and smooth.
6. Scrape the batter into the baking pan and level the batter with a spatula.
7. Slide the baking pan into Rack Position 1, select Convection Bake set the temperature to 325°F (163°C), and set time to 20 minutes.
8. After 15 minutes, remove the pan from the oven. Check the doneness. Return the pan to the oven and continue cooking.
9. When done, a toothpick inserted in the center should come out clean.
10. Invert the cake on a cooling rack and allow it to cool for 15 minutes before slicing to serve.

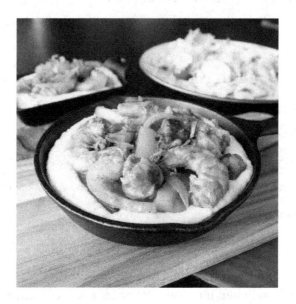

Serves: 4

Ingredients:

- 1 tablespoon Sriracha sauce

- 1 teaspoon Worcestershire sauce

- 2 tablespoons sweet chili sauce

- ¾ cup mayonnaise

- 1 egg, beaten

- 1 cup panko bread crumbs

- 1 pound (454 g) raw shrimp, shelled and deveined, rinsed and drained

- Lime wedges, for serving

- Cooking spray

Directions:

1. Spritz the air fryer basket with cooking spray.

2. Combine the Sriracha sauce, Worcestershire sauce, chili sauce, and mayo in a bowl. Stir to mix well. Reserve ⅓ cup of the mixture as the dipping sauce.

3. Combine the remaining sauce mixture with the beaten egg. Stir to mix well. Put the panko in a separate bowl.

4. Dredge the shrimp in the sauce mixture first, then into the panko. Roll the shrimp to coat well. Shake the excess off.

5. Place the shrimp in the basket, then spritz with cooking spray.

6. Put the air fryer basket on the baking pan and slide into Rack Position 2, select Air Fry, set temperature to 360°F (182°C), and set time to 10 minutes.

7. Flip the shrimp halfway through the cooking time.

8. When cooking is complete, the shrimp should be opaque.

9. Remove the shrimp from the oven and serve with a reserve sauce mixture and squeeze the lime wedges over.

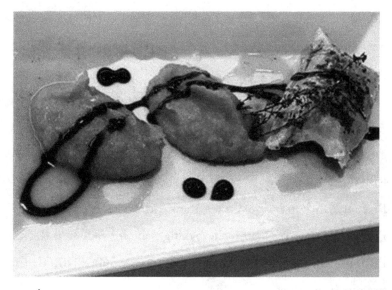

Serves: 4

Ingredients

- large salmon trout filleted on 4 pieces, the carcasses save for the rear
- 50 g Celery, finely chopped
- 50 g Carrot, finely chopped
- 50 g Leek, finely chopped
- stripsPeel the orange peel, wide, 2 times with the peeler
- Parsley
- Tarragon
- Some orange zest
- 200 ml fish stock
- 60 ml Vinegar, light, sweet (apple balsamic vinegar)
- Peppercorns, white

- Allspice
- 40 ml White wine
- 60 ml Noilly Prat
- tbsp. Coconut milk, the solid ingredient
- 2 cm ginger
- 2 stems of lemongrass, in pieces
- Kaffir lime leaves
- large ones Sweet potato
- 2 m. In size Potato
- Rear
- Salt and pepper

Directions

1. First, fillet the salmon trout and peel off the skin. Pull out the bones with a pair of fish tongs and lightly season the fillets on the inside with salt and pepper. Then cover the inside with parsley, tarragon, and orange zest and set the fillets aside.

2. Bring the fish stock to the boil with vinegar, white wine, Noilly Prat, coconut milk, the spices (allspice, pepper, ginger, lemongrass, kaffir lime leaves), and the fish carcasses and reduce them by about 15 - 20 minutes.

3. Meanwhile, lightly fry the vegetable strips with the orange peel in a little clarified butter and season with salt and pepper.

4. Put some vegetables in suitable vacuum bags, put a fillet on each, and pour some stock. Then seal the bags with a vacuum device.

5. Peel the sweet potatoes and potatoes cut them into pieces and steam them in the steamer for about 30 minutes. Then press through a potato press and season with a thickened stock, salt, and pepper, and keep warm.

6. Cook the fish fillets in a water bath at 56 ° C for 18 minutes.

7. Place a sweet potato purée on preheated plates, cut open a sack, drape the contents on the mirrors and cover with fish stock. Decorate as desired.

Index

A

B

C

E

F

G

H

J

K

L

M

R

S

T

Cooking Conversion Chart

TEMPERATURE		WEIGHT	
FAHRENHEIT	**CELSIUS**	**IMPERIAL**	**METRIC**
100 °F	37 °C	1/2 oz	15 g
150 °F	65 °C	1 oz	29 g
200 °F	93 °C	2 oz	57 g
250 °F	121 °C	3 oz	85 g
300 °F	150 °C	4 oz	113 g
325 °F	160 °C	5 oz	141 g
350 °F	180 °C	6 oz	170 g
375 °F	190 °C	8 oz	227 g
400 °F	200 °C	10 oz	283 g
425 °F	220 °C	12 oz	340 g
450 °F	230 °C	13 oz	369 g
500 °F	260 °C	14 oz	397 g
525 °F	270 °C	15 oz	425 g
550 °F	288 °C	1 lb	453 g

MEASUREMENT			
CUP	ONCES	MILLILITERS	TABLESPOON
1/16 cup	1/2 oz	15 ml	1
1/8 cup	1 oz	30 ml	3
1/4 cup	2 oz	59 ml	4
1/3 cup	2.5 oz	79 ml	5.5
3/8 cup	3 oz	90 ml	6
1/2 cup	4 oz	118 ml	8
2/3 cup	5 oz	158 ml	11
3/4 cup	6 oz	177 ml	12
1 cup	8 oz	240 ml	16
2 cup	16 oz	480 ml	32
4 cup	32 oz	960 ml	64
5 cup	40 oz	1180 ml	80
6 cup	48 oz	1420 ml	96
8 cup	64 oz	1895 ml	128

CPSIA information can be obtained
at www.ICGtesting.com
Printed in the USA
BVHW091119220621
610208BV00002B/66